HEALTHY ATLANTIC DISHES

Explore over 20 flavorful Atlantic dishes medically beneficial to health and healthy slim

Theresa Arlene

Table of contents

Introduction

Atlantic cuisine is a unique style of cooking that encompasses the food and flavours of the North Atlantic region. Its origin dates all the way back to the Viking era, when Norse fishermen and explorers settled along northern Europe's coastlines. This ancient cuisine draws upon the region's rich natural resources of seafood, grains, dairy products, and vegetables.

At its core, Atlantic cuisine is all about celebrating the bounty of the sea. Classic dishes often incorporate fresh seafood like cod, haddock, halibut, and mollusks. Atlantic dishes also feature regional species such as herring, mussels, scallops, squid, salmon, and lobster. Popular seafood preparations also include smoked or pickled fish.

Atlantic cuisine's land-based ingredients are equally delish, including grains like barley, wheat and oats, and root vegetables like potatoes, beets, and carrots. You can also find hearty staples like pork, beef, lamb, chicken, and game birds.

If you're a fan of sauces, then Atlantic cuisine won't disappoint. Popular local sauces that pair well with seafood include creamy ramp butter, lemon-dill mayonnaise, and white or redwine butter sauces.

Health Benefits

First and foremost, the Atlantic region is abundant with fresh seafood, vegetables, and a variety of grains. These foods are all loaded with essential vitamins and minerals, and the diet of an Atlantic-dweller typically consists of copious amounts of these nutrient-rich foods. As a result, Atlantic residents tend to have higher intakes of those vitamins and minerals, which can promote healthy growth and development.

The health benefits of Atlantic dishes are vast and varied when considering the many dishes that can be made and served in this geographic region. From hearty stews, rustic seafood dishes, fresh salads and indulgent desserts, the Atlantic region's cuisine has something for everyone.

Fresh seafood is a staple of the Atlantic diet, and, when combined with healthy side dishes, can offer a range of health benefits. For instance, many types of seafood, like salmon, are rich in omega-3 fatty acids, which are known to reduce the risk of stroke, heart disease, depression and cognitive decline. Other seafood dishes, such as sole and cod, are rich sources of iodine and vitamin D, which can help boost immunity and reduce inflammation in the body.

The abundance of vegetables in the Atlantic region has made it possible to produce a range of health-promoting dishes with unique textures and flavors. For example, the hearty vegan stew "Falkandean Beans and Greens" is a perfect example of a nutrient-rich dish. Additionally, the classic Atlantic salad dish, Caesar salad, is packed with greens and provides a massive amount of vitamins and minerals.

The Atlantic region is also home to many delicious dishes that incorporate whole grains. Products like quinoa, oats, barley and corn are all staples in the area and can be readily found in various recipes. These grains are all packed with dietary fiber and essential vitamins and minerals. Fiber can help regulate digestion, reduce cholesterol levels and keep you feeling full for longer.

Atlantic dishes are also known for their use of various types of protein sources, from lean proteins like chicken breast, to fish like cod and tuna. Eating lean proteins is necessary for maintaining optimal health and the Atlantic region's cuisine provides a great source of these important nutritional components needed for a balanced diet.

In addition to the vast nutritional benefits associated with the Atlantic region's cuisine, many of the dishes are also surprisingly low in calories. For example, the hearty stew "Falkandean Beans and Greens" is packed with nutrients but contains only around 300 calories. Combining dishes like this with other healthy options allows you to enjoy a well-balanced meal without compromising your weight-loss goals.

In conclusion, the Atlantic region's cuisine offers a variety of health benefits that can fit into any diet. From fresh seafood, to heartwarming stews, to indulgent desserts – it's all packed with the key vitamins and minerals needed to maintain good health. What's more, many of these dishes are surprisingly low in calories, allowing you to enjoy healthy dishes without compromising your weight-loss goals. All in all, Atlantic dishes can provide a well-rounded, nutritious diet that is sure to promote better overall health.

ATLANTIC FOOD

RECIPES

Fish And Chips

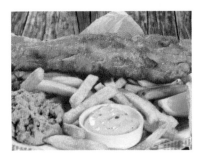

Fish and chips is a traditional British dish consisting of fried battered fish and thin cut chips (french fries). The fish is usually cod, haddock, or plaice, and is dipped in a batter that consists of flour, eggs, milk, and occasionally other ingredients. The chips are usually served with malt vinegar, ketchup, and various sauces. The dish is normally served in a paper wrapping to help keep it warm.

Ingredients:

- ➢ Vegetable oil, for frying
- ➢ 1 cup all-purpose flour
- ➢ 2 tsp baking powder
- ➢ ½ tsp garlic powder
- ➢ 2 tsp paprika
- ➢ Salt and pepper, to taste
- ➢ 1 cup (240 ml) beer

- 1 pound (455 g) cod fillet, cut into strips

- 1 cup (50 g) panko breadcrumbs

- 2-3 potatoes, cut into fry shapes

Instructions:

- Heat the vegetable oil in a large skillet over medium-high heat.

- Meanwhile, in a large bowl, whisk together the flour, baking powder, garlic powder, paprika, salt and pepper.

- Slowly whisk in the beer until the batter is smooth.

- Dip each piece of fish into the batter and then roll in the breadcrumbs to coat.

- Carefully add the coated fish strips to the hot oil and fry until golden-brown and cooked through, about 3-4 minutes.

- Remove fish and transfer to a paper towel-lined plate.

- Repeat with the potatoes, adding them to the hot oil and frying until golden and crispy, about 5 minutes.

- Serve the fish and chips with your favorite dipping sauce. Enjoy!

Crème Brulee

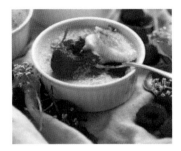

Crème brulee (or crème brulee) is a popular French custard dessert consisting of a rich custard base topped with a contrasting layer of hard caramelized sugar. The combination of the creamy custard and crisp, caramelized topping make for a delightful sweet treat. The custard is traditionally flavored with vanilla, but variations can include other ingredients such as orange zest, lavender, or rum. Crème brulee is often served with a selection of fresh fruit or a dollop of whipped cream, but can also be enjoyed on its own.

Ingredients:

- ➤ 4 cups heavy cream
- ➤ 1 cup granulated sugar
- ➤ 6 large egg yolks
- ➤ 1 teaspoon vanilla extract
- ➤ ¼ cup packed light brown sugar

Instructions:

- Preheat oven to 325F.
- In a saucepan, heat cream and granulated sugar over medium heat until hot, but not boiling.
- In a medium bowl, whisk egg yolks until smooth.
- Slowly pour the hot cream mixture into the egg yolks, whisking constantly.
- Add the vanilla extract and whisk to combine.
- Pour the mixture into 4-6 oven-safe ramekins, filling each about halfway.
- Place the ramekins in a baking dish and fill with enough hot water to come halfway up the sides of the ramekins.
- Bake for 45 minutes to an hour or until the custard is set.
- Carefully remove the ramekins from the baking dish and allow to cool for 15 minutes.
- Sprinkle a thin layer of brown sugar over each custard and, using a torch, melt the sugar until it forms a golden caramelized crust. Serve immediately.

Gravlax

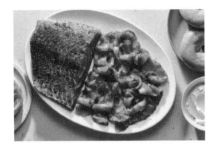

Gravlax is a classic Atlantic dish of cured salmon. This dish has its origin in the Norse days of the Viking era, when fishermen would resort to curing salmon to preserve the fish for longer periods of time. Although the curing process was abandoned when modern refrigeration became available, the tradition of gravlax is still enjoyed throughout the North Atlantic region.

Ingredients:

- ➤ 2 lb. salmon fillet, skin and pin bones removed
- ➤ ½ cup sea salt
- ➤ ½ cup light brown sugar
- ➤ ¼ cup cracked juniper berries
- ➤ 2 tsp. freshly ground white pepper
- ➤ ¼ cup fresh dill, finely chopped

Instructions:

- Line a large shallow container with plastic wrap. Lay the salmon fillet in the center of the container, and sprinkle with the salt, sugar, juniper berries, and white pepper.

- Sprinkle the chopped dill over the top of the salmon, then cover the entire top surface of the salmon with a generous layer of the remaining ingredients.

- Wrap the salmon tightly with the plastic wrap, pressing down on the ingredients to ensure even distribution. Refrigerate for approximately 24 hours.

- Garnish with extra fresh dill, if desired, and serve over a bed of fresh greens.

Clams Casino

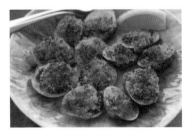

Clams casino is a dish made from chopped clams, bacon, and a creamy sauce made from butter, flour, and cream. It usually has garlic, parsley, and other spices. It is usually served over linguini pasta or topped with breadcrumbs. The dish originated in Rhode Island and is popular in the northeastern United States. It can also be served as an appetizer.

Ingredients:

- 1 lb. fresh clams
- 3 tbsp butter
- 3 cloves garlic, minced
- 1/4 cup dry white wine
- 2 tbsp panko breadcrumbs
- 2 tbsp grated Parmesan cheese
- 1 tsp lemon zest
- Salt and pepper, to taste
- 1/4 cup fresh parsley, finely chopped

- ➢ 1 lemon, cut into wedges

Instructions:

- ✦ Preheat oven to 350°F and butter a baking dish.

- ✦ Rinse the clams well and set aside.

- ✦ Heat the butter in a large skillet over medium heat. When melted, add the garlic and sauté until fragrant, about 1 minute.

- ✦ Add the white wine and simmer until reduced slightly, about 2 minutes.

- ✦ Add the clams, cover the skillet and steam until the clams open, about 5-7 minutes. Discard any clams that do not open.

- ✦ Transfer the clams and garlic to the prepared baking dish.

- ✦ Combine the panko, Parmesan cheese, lemon zest, salt and pepper in a small bowl.

- ✦ Sprinkle the mixture evenly over the top of the clams.

- ✦ Bake until the topping is golden and the clams are cooked through, about 10 minutes.

- ✦ Garnish with fresh parsley and serve with lemon wedges. Enjoy!

Fish Cakes with Mustard Butter Sauce

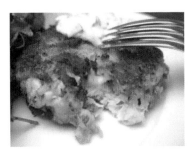

This classic Atlantic recipe is a favourite throughout the coastal regions of the North Atlantic. Made with fish and potato, and served with a mustard butter sauce, this dish is as flavourful as it is economical. To best capture the flavours of Atlantic cuisine, use locally procured fish, preferably cod or haddock.

Ingredients:

- 1 lb. cod or haddock fillets, skin removed and diced fine
- 1 lb potatoes, peeled and diced
- 1/3 cup minced green onion
- ½ cup bread crumbs
- 1 egg, lightly beaten
- 2 tbsp. butter
- 1 tsp. dried dill
- Dash of sea salt
- Dash of ground black pepper

- ➢ 2 tbsp. olive oil

Mustard Butter Sauce:

- ➢ 2 tbsp. butter
- ➢ 2 cloves garlic, minced
- ➢ ¼ cup white wine
- ➢ 2 tbsp. Dijon mustard
- ➢ 1 tsp. dried dill

Instructions:

- In a large bowl, combine the diced fish, potatoes, green onion, bread crumbs, egg, butter, dill, salt, and pepper. Mix thoroughly, making sure all ingredients are evenly distributed.
- Form the fish mixture into cakes about ½ inch thick.
- Heat the olive oil in a large skillet over medium-high heat. Place the cakes in the pan, and cook for about 3 minutes per side, or until the cakes are golden brown.
- While the cakes are cooking, prepare the mustard butter sauce. In a small saucepan, melt the butter over medium heat. Add the garlic, and cook for 1-2 minutes. Deglaze the pan with the white wine, and

stir in the mustard and dill. Allow the sauce to reduce and thicken for about 5 minutes.

🔸 Serve the fish cakes with the mustard butter sauce.

Lobster Roll

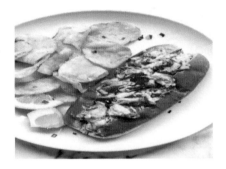

A lobster roll is a type of sandwich typically filled with lobster meat, mayonnaise, and other seasonings such as celery and onion. The lobster is usually chopped and the sandwich is served on a steamed and buttered toasted roll. This dish is originally from New England, although variations can be found throughout the US and Canada.

Ingredients:

- 1/2 lb cooked lobster meat
- 1/4 cup mayonnaise
- 2 tablespoons celery, chopped
- 2 tablespoons green onion, chopped
- 1 tablespoon fresh parsley, chopped
- 2 tablespoons lemon juice
- 1/4 teaspoon salt
- 1/8 teaspoon black pepper
- 4 hot dog buns
- 1/4 cup unsalted butter, melted

Instructions:

- In a medium bowl, mix together the lobster meat, mayonnaise, celery, green onion, parsley, lemon juice, salt, and pepper.
- To assemble the rolls, place a bun on a work surface. Spread 2 tablespoons of the lobster mixture on the bottom of each bun. Place the top bun on and press lightly.
- Heat a large skillet over medium-high heat.

- Brush one side of each bun with melted butter and place the bun buttered side down in the skillet. Cook for 2 minutes, or until golden brown.

- Brush the top of each bun with butter and flip them over. Cook for an additional 2 minutes, or until golden brown.

- Serve hot with your favorite seafood sides and enjoy!

Fish Cakes

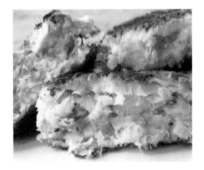

Fish cakes are patties made from fish, bread crumbs, and other ingredients such as onion, bell pepper, parsley, and spices. They can be served as appetizers, entrées, or snacks. Fish cakes may be deep-fried or pan-fried and can be served as a sandwich or on a salad. They can be eaten hot or cold.

Ingredients:

- ➢ 2 pounds of fresh cod fillets, skinless and boneless
- ➢ 2 large potatoes, peeled and cut into ½-inch cubes
- ➢ 2 tablespoons of minced fresh parsley
- ➢ 2 tablespoons of minced fresh dill
- ➢ 2 large eggs, beaten
- ➢ ½ cup of all-purpose flour
- ➢ ¼ cup of panko breadcrumbs
- ➢ 2 teaspoons of salt
- ➢ ½ teaspoon of ground black pepper
- ➢ 2 tablespoons of olive oil
- ➢ ½ cup of mayonnaise
- ➢ 1 tablespoon of Dijon mustard
- ➢ 2 tablespoons of freshly squeezed lemon juice

Instructions:

- ♣ Place the cod fillets in a large saucepan and cover with cold water.

- Bring to a boil over high heat and cook for 4 to 5 minutes, or until the fish is cooked through and flakes easily with a fork.

- Remove the fish from the water and place onto a cutting board. Discard the cooking liquid.

- Flake the cooked cod into small pieces and place into a large mixing bowl.

- Add the potatoes, parsley, dill, eggs, flour, breadcrumbs, salt, and pepper to the bowl and mix together until well combined.

- Using wet hands, form the mixture into small patties.

- Heat the oil in a large non-stick skillet over medium-high heat.

- Add the fish cakes to the skillet and cook for 3 to 5 minutes per side, or until golden-brown and crispy.

- Remove the fish cakes from the skillet and transfer to a plate lined with paper towels to absorb any excess oil.

- In a small bowl, mix together the mayonnaise, Dijon mustard, and lemon juice.

- Serve the fish cakes with the flavored mayonnaise. Enjoy!

Seafood Chowder

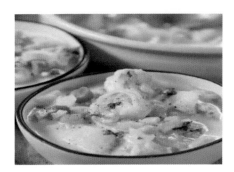

Seafood chowder is a thick, creamy soup or stew made with various types of seafood and full of robust flavors. It typically features a base of creamy milk or cream, potatoes, onions, celery, and herbs such as parsley, thyme, or rosemary. The soup also commonly includes white fish, clams, shrimp, or other types of seafood. It is often accompanied by freshly cooked crackers, oyster crackers, or toasted bread. The dish is typically served steaming hot and can be enjoyed as a main course with a side dish, such as a salad or roll.

Ingredients:

> - 2 tablespoons oil
> - 1 small onion, diced
> - 4 cloves garlic, minced
> - ½ cup celery, diced
> - 3 tablespoons tomato paste
> - 2 tablespoons all-purpose flour

- ➤ 4 cups fish or vegetable stock
- ➤ 2 medium potatoes, peeled and diced
- ➤ 2 cups diced carrots
- ➤ ½ pound white fish (such as cod or haddock)
- ➤ ½ pound shrimp
- ➤ ½ teaspoon dried thyme
- ➤ 1 bay leaf
- ➤ ½ teaspoon salt
- ➤ ¼ teaspoon white pepper
- ➤ ½ cup heavy cream
- ➤ ½ cup frozen corn
- ➤ ½ cup frozen green peas
- ➤ 2 tablespoons chopped fresh parsley

Instructions:

- ✦ Heat the oil in a large pot over medium-high heat. Add the onion, garlic, and celery and cook until soft and fragrant, about 5 minutes.
- ✦ Add the tomato paste and flour and cook for 1 minute, stirring constantly.

- Add in the stock, potatoes, carrots, fish, shrimp, thyme, bay leaf, salt and pepper. Bring to a boil, reduce the heat and simmer until the potatoes and

- carrots are tender, about 15 minutes.

- Stir in the cream, corn, peas, and parsley. Simmer for an additional 5 minutes.

- Discard the bay leaf before serving. Serve hot. Enjoy!

Fish Tacos

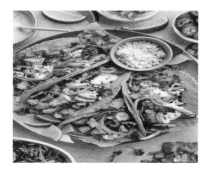

Fish tacos are a Mexican-style dish comprised of a corn or flour tortilla, filled with lightly fried or grilled fish, and topped with shredded cabbage, pico de gallo, and a creamy sauce such as sour cream, chipotle mayo, or ranch. Other variations may include avocado, guacamole, limes, pickled onions, or cilantro. The tacos can be served as individual tacos, or arranged side-by-side for a larger portion. Fish tacos are typically served with sides such as chips, salsa, and/or refried beans.

Ingredients:

- 2 lbs. skinless, boneless cod fillets
- 4 tablespoons vegetable oil
- 1 teaspoon garlic powder
- 2 teaspoons chili powder
- 1 cup all-purpose flour
- 2 teaspoons ground cumin
- 2 tablespoons chopped fresh cilantro
- 2 cups Mexican-style panko bread crumbs
- 8 small soft taco shells
- 2 cups Lime Cabbage Slaw
- ½ cup sour cream

Instructions:

- Preheat oven to 425 degrees F.
- Cut cod into 2-inch pieces, and set aside.

- In a shallow dish, mix together the vegetable oil, garlic powder, chili powder, flour and cumin.

- Toss the cod pieces in the mixture until evenly coated.

- Place the panko bread crumbs into another shallow dish.

- Dip each piece of cod in the panko, and then place on a lightly greased baking sheet.

- Bake the cod pieces in the preheated oven for 15 minutes, or until cooked through and golden brown.

- To assemble the tacos, fill each shell with a piece of fish, top with Lime Slaw, and a dollop of sour cream.

Boiled Lobster

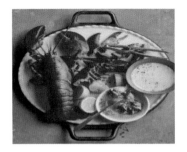

Boiled lobster is a seafood dish that is prepared by cooking a lobster in boiling water. Lobsters that are used for boiling can be either freshly caught or thawed from previously frozen lobsters. Boiled lobster will typically be lightly salted to bring out its natural flavor. The result of boiling is a lobster with a delicately sweet flavor that pairs well with a variety of side dishes. Most boiled lobsters can be eaten as-is or with melted butter, lemon wedges, and sauces.

Ingredients:

- 2-4 live lobsters
- Water
- Salt
- Butter

Instructions:

- Fill a large pot with enough water to cover the lobsters completely.

- Add 2 tablespoons of salt for every quart of water.

- Bring the water to a rolling boil.

- Carefully add the live lobsters into the boiling water.

- Boil for 11-13 minutes, depending on the size of the lobster.

- Remove the lobsters from the pot using tongs, and place in ice water.

- When lobsters have cooled, twist off the claws, remove the tail and crack the shell open.

- Serve with melted butter or your favorite dipping sauce. Enjoy!

Fried Clams

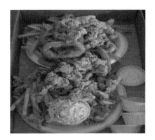

Fried clams are usually made from the soft-shell clam, which are shucked and dredged in seasoned flour before being deep fried. The coating is typically a combination of cornmeal, flour, or breadcrumbs, which give the fried clams a crunchy texture. They are usually served with tartar sauce on the side and sometimes a slice of lemon. This dish is a classic seafood favorite, popular on the east coast of the United States.

Ingredients:

- 1 pound small fresh clams
- 1 cup all-purpose flour
- 1 teaspoon baking powder
- 1/2 teaspoon kosher salt
- 1/4 teaspoon freshly ground black pepper
- 1/2 teaspoon Old Bay Seasoning
- 1 large egg
- 1/2 cup milk
- 2 tablespoons unsalted butter, melted
- Vegetable oil, for deep-frying
- Lemon wedges, for serving

Instructions:

- Rinse the clams under cold running water and place them in a colander to drain.

- In a shallow bowl, whisk together the flour, baking powder, salt, pepper, and Old Bay seasoning. In a separate bowl, beat the egg and then whisk in the milk and melted butter.

- Dip each clam in the egg mixture, turning to coat. Allow the excess to drip off and then dredge the clams in the flour mixture.

- Heat oil in a deep-fryer or large pot to 375°F. Working in batches, add the clams to the hot oil and fry until golden brown, about 3 minutes. Remove with a slotted spoon and drain on paper towels.

- Serve immediately with lemon wedges. Enjoy!

Oysters Rockefeller

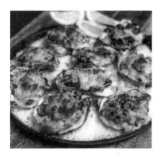

Oysters Rockefeller is a classic French-American dish made of oysters on the half-shell baked with a stuffing of butter, parsley, breadcrumbs, and other herbs such as chervil, tarragon, and fennel. It is often topped with an herbed butter sauce and/or a variety of cheeses, and cooked until hot and bubbly before serving. The dish is named after John D. Rockefeller, the American businessman and philanthropist, and is thought to have been created at Antoine's restaurant in New Orleans, Louisiana.

Ingredients:

- 2 dozen small to medium oysters on the half shell
- 2 tablespoons butter
- 4 green onions, finely chopped
- 1/3 cup finely chopped celery
- 3 tablespoons freshly squeezed lemon juice
- 2 tablespoons Worcestershire sauce
- ¼ teaspoon fine sea salt
- Freshly ground black pepper
- 2 tablespoons anise liqueur (optional)
- 2 tablespoons freshly grated Parmesan cheese
- 3 tablespoons fresh parsley leaves, chopped
- 2 tablespoons plain dried breadcrumbs
- 2 tablespoons freshly grated Pecorino Romano cheese

Instructions:

- Preheat oven to 400°F (205°C).

- Place oysters on a baking sheet in their half shells.

- In a medium skillet, melt the butter over medium heat and add the green onions, celery, lemon juice, Worcestershire sauce, salt, and pepper. Cook for about 3 minutes, stirring frequently, until the vegetables soften.

- Add the anise liqueur, if using, and cook for another minute.

- Add the Parmesan cheese, parsley, and breadcrumbs, and mix until well blended.

- Spoon approximately one tablespoon of the mixture over each of the oysters.

- Sprinkle Pecorino Romano cheese over the oysters.

- Bake for 10-15 minutes, or until the oysters are cooked and the topping is golden brown.

- Serve hot. Enjoy!

Salmon Fillet

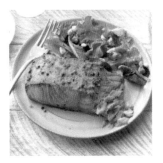

A Salmon fillet is a boneless cut of salmon, typically cut from the back of the fish. Salmon fillets are lean and subtle in flavor, with firm, succulent and medium-textured flesh. Salmon fillets generally have a pink to orange color, but can also depending on the variety of salmon. They are a great source of omega-3 fatty acids, protein, potassium, Vitamin A, and Vitamin D.

Ingredients:

- 4 (6-ounce) salmon fillets
- 2 tablespoons olive oil
- 2 tablespoons fresh lemon juice
- 1 teaspoon kosher salt
- 1/4 teaspoon freshly ground black pepper
- 1/4 cup chopped fresh parsley
- 2 tablespoons chopped fresh dill

> 1/4 cup dry white wine

Instructions:

- Preheat oven to 400 degrees F.

- Place salmon fillets in a baking dish and drizzle with olive oil, lemon juice, salt, and pepper.

- Bake for 10 minutes, or until fish is cooked through.

- Meanwhile, mix together the parsley, dill, and wine in a small bowl.

- When done, remove salmon from the oven and spoon the herb mixture over the top.

- Serve with your favorite sides and enjoy!

Mussels Fra Diavolo

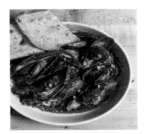

Mussels fra diavolo is a classic Italian seafood dish that consists of mussels cooked in a spicy tomato sauce. The sauce typically includes tomatoes, garlic, onions, and red pepper flakes. The dish is typically served over spaghetti or other pasta, and its name comes from the Italian phrase "diablo", which translates roughly to "devil". Mussels fra diavolo is a simple and flavorful dish that is sure to spice up any seafood night.

Ingredients:

- 2 tablespoons olive oil
- 6 cloves garlic, minced
- ½ teaspoon red pepper flakes
- ¼ teaspoon black pepper
- ½ teaspoon dried oregano
- 2 (14-ounce) cans diced tomatoes
- ¼ cup white wine
- ½ cup chopped fresh parsley

- ¼ cup chopped fresh basil

- 2 pounds mussels, scrubbed and debearded

- Grated Parmesan cheese, for garnish

Instructions:

- In a large pot over medium heat, heat the olive oil. Add the garlic, red pepper flakes, black pepper, and oregano. Sauté until the garlic is lightly browned, about 1 minute.

- Add the tomatoes and wine and bring to a simmer. Reduce the heat to low and simmer for 10 minutes.

- Add the parsley and basil, and stir to combine.

- Add the mussels, cover, and cook until the mussels open, about 5 minutes. Discard any unopened mussels.

- To serve, ladle the mussels and sauce into a serving bowl. Sprinkle with Parmesan cheese. Enjoy!

Seafood Paella

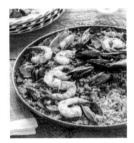

Seafood paella is a popular Spanish dish made with a combination of saffron-infused rice, vegetables, and seafood. It traditionally includes shrimp, mussels, and squid, but other local seafood such as crab, clams, or fish can also be used. It is usually flavored with herbs and spices such as garlic, smoked paprika, saffron, and parsley. It is usually served with a side of allioli (garlic mayonnaise) for an added burst of flavor. It is a hearty, flavorful, and incredibly satisfying dish.

Ingredients:

- 2 cups paella rice
- 4-5 cups chicken broth
- ½ cup olive oil
- 2 cloves garlic, minced
- 1 large onion, chopped
- 4 ounces chopped cured chorizo sausage
- 1 large red bell pepper, diced

- 2 cups diced ripe tomatoes
- ½ teaspoon saffron threads
- ½ teaspoon smoked paprika
- 1 teaspoon salt
- ½ teaspoon freshly ground black pepper
- ½ pound raw prawns
- ½ pound mussels
- ½ pound squid, sliced into rings
- 2 cups cooked white beans
- 2 tablespoons chopped fresh parsley
- Lemon wedges, for serving

Instructions:

- Preheat oven to 350°F.
- In a large ovenproof pan, heat the olive oil over medium heat.
- Add the garlic and onions and cook until softened, about 5 minutes.
- Add the chorizo sausage and cook for an additional 3-4 minutes.
- Add the red bell pepper, tomatoes, saffron, paprika, salt, and pepper and cook for another 2 minutes.

- Add the paella rice and chicken broth to the pan and stir to combine. Bring to a simmer and cook until liquid is absorbed, stirring occasionally.

- Add the prawns, mussels, squid, white beans, and parsley to the pan and stir to combine.

- Transfer the pan to the preheated oven and bake uncovered for about 15 minutes.

- Remove from the oven and let stand for 10 minutes before serving.

- Serve with lemon wedges and enjoy!

Maple-Glazed Salmon

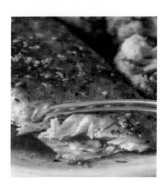

Maple-glazed salmon is a type of fish dish made by coating salmon with a sweet and savory glaze made of maple syrup, soy sauce, ginger, and garlic. The resulting fish has a slightly crispy outside layer with a sweet and tangy taste. It is best served over a bed of brown rice or steamed vegetables.

Ingredients:

- 4 (4-ounce) salmon fillets
- 1/4 cup pure maple syrup
- 1 tablespoon extra-virgin olive oil
- 2 teaspoons Dijon mustard
- 1/4 teaspoon sea salt
- 1/8 teaspoon freshly ground black pepper

Instructions:

- Preheat oven to 425°F.

- Place salmon fillets on a baking sheet lined with parchment paper.

- In a small bowl, whisk together maple syrup, olive oil, mustard, salt, and pepper.

- Brush the mixture over the top of each salmon fillet.

- Bake in preheated oven for 12 minutes, or until cooked through.

- Serve over a bed of greens, with lemon wedges, if desired. Enjoy!

Escargot

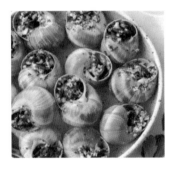

Escargot is a French culinary dish consisting of cooked land snails. It is typically served as an appetizer in garlic-butter sauce. Escargot is known for its firm, chewy texture and distinctive flavour. In some countries, including the U.S., the snails used are generally escaped pet snails, as true escargot is illegal to import.

Ingredients:

- ➤ 24 Escargot snails
- ➤ 2 cloves of garlic, finely chopped
- ➤ ½ cup of butter
- ➤ ¼ cup of dry white wine
- ➤ 2 tablespoons of chopped parsley
- ➤ 2 tablespoons of chopped shallots or onions
- ➤ ½ teaspoon of freshly ground black pepper
- ➤ ¼ teaspoon of sea salt

Instructions:

- ✦ Preheat your oven to 375°F (190°C).
- ✦ Place the snails in a large oven-safe baking dish.
- ✦ In a medium bowl, mix together the garlic, butter, white wine, parsley, shallots (or onions), black pepper, and salt.
- ✦ Pour this mixture over the snails, and make sure all the snails are coated.

- Bake in the preheated oven for about 20 minutes, or until the snails are cooked through.

- Serve hot with crunchy bread.

Oyster On The Half Shell

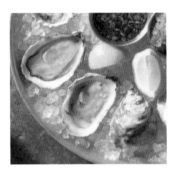

Oysters on the half shell are oysters that have been shucked, meaning their two shells have been separated and the oyster has been removed from inside. The oyster is served in one half of its shell, usually with a dash of lemon juice and hot sauce on top. These oysters are often served as appetizers or snacks, or as part of a seafood platter. They are also eaten raw or steamed

Ingredients:

- 3-4 dozen live oysters
- 2 lemons, juiced
- 2 tablespoons chopped fresh parsley
- 2 tablespoons minced shallots
- 1 tablespoon extra-virgin olive oil
- 2 tablespoons white wine
- Salt and pepper to taste

Instructions:

- Place the oysters flat side up on a baking sheet. Put them into the oven and bake at 350°F for 10 minutes.
- Remove the oysters from the oven and shuck the shells, being careful not to puncture the top and bottom.
- Place the oysters on a plate and spoon the juice on top.
- Squeeze the lemons over the plate and sprinkle the parsley, shallots, olive oil, and white wine over the plate.
- Sprinkle salt and pepper to taste. Serve with bread, crackers, and lemon wedges. Enjoy!

Soft Shell Crab Dish

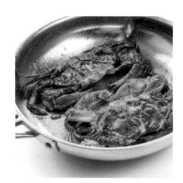

Soft shell crab is a popular seafood dish made with freshly caught crabs. The crab is lightly battered and deep-fried until it is golden brown and crispy. The soft shell of the crab remains intact giving it a unique texture and taste. It is typically served with a lemon wedge, tartar sauce, and a cold crisp salad. Soft shell crabs are often used in sushi, salads, tacos, and other Asian-inspired dishes.

Ingredients:

- 2 Soft Shell Crabs
- 2 Tbsp Olive Oil
- 1/2 cup White Wine
- 2 cloves Garlic, minced
- 1/4 cup Shallots, sliced
- 1 Tbsp Chopped Parsley
- Salt & Pepper to taste

> Lemon Wedges for garnish

Instructions:

- Heat the olive oil in a large skillet over medium-high heat.

- Add the soft shell crabs to the skillet and cook until golden brown on both sides, about 4 minutes per side.

- Reduce the heat to medium-low, add the white wine, garlic, shallots, and parsley.

- Simmer for a few minutes until the sauce has reduced and thickened.

- Season with salt and pepper to taste and serve with lemon wedges. Enjoy!

Calamari

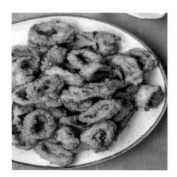

Calamari is a type of seafood dish typically made from squid. It is usually fried or served in a spicy sauce. Calamari has a soft texture and a mild flavor, and often comes lightly breaded for added crunchiness. It is a popular fried appetizer in Mediterranean-style restaurants. In some regions, it is made by battering and deep-frying squid rings.

Ingredients:

> ➤ 2 lbs whole calamari, cleaned and cut into 1-inch rings

> ➤ ¼ cup olive oil

> ➤ 2 cloves garlic, minced

> ➤ 2 tablespoons fresh lemon juice

> ➤ 2 tablespoons chopped fresh parsley

> ➤ 1 teaspoon dried oregano

> ➤ ¼ teaspoon sea salt

> ➤ ¼ teaspoon freshly ground pepper

- ¼ cup all-purpose flour

- ½ cup dry white wine

- 2 tablespoons butter

- 2 tablespoons capers

- Lemon wedges for serving

Instructions:

- In a large bowl, combine the calamari, olive oil, garlic, lemon juice, parsley, oregano, salt, and pepper. Mix until the calamari is evenly coated.

- Preheat a large skillet over medium-high heat.

- Place the flour in a shallow dish. Dredge the calamari rings in the flour, shaking off any excess. Reserve the remaining flour.

- Add 2 tablespoons of butter to the skillet and swirl to coat.

- Add the calamari to the skillet and cook for 4 minutes, turning once, until the calamari is lightly browned and cooked through.

- Reduce heat to medium. Add the wine to the skillet and swirl to combine.

- Add the remaining butter and the capers. Cook for 3 minutes, stirring occasionally until the sauce has thickened.

- Add the reserved flour and stir to combine. Cook for 1 minute, stirring constantly, until the sauce has thickened.

- Divide the calamari between plates and serve with lemon wedges. Enjoy!

Scones

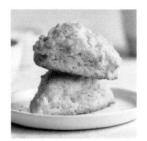

Scones are small, round pastries that are made by combining flour, butter, milk, baking powder, and sugar. They can be either sweet or savory, and are usually served with jam, cream, or butter. The traditional shape is round and flat, but other shapes, including triangles, are also popular. Scones are often served at a tea or brunch, alongside tea sandwiches, tea cakes, and other items.

Ingredients:

- ¾ cup melted butter
- ¼ cup white sugar
- 2 eggs
- 2 cups all-purpose flour
- ½ cup whole wheat flour
- 4 teaspoons baking powder
- ½ teaspoon salt
- 1 teaspoon vanilla extract
- 1 ½ cups heavy cream

Instructions:

- Preheat the oven to 425 degrees Fahrenheit.
- In a large bowl, mix together the melted butter and white sugar until well-combined.
- Whisk in the eggs until everything is evenly blended.
- In a separate bowl, combine the all-purpose flour, whole wheat flour, baking powder, and salt.
- Gradually add the dry ingredients to the wet ingredients, stirring until just combined. Do not overmix.

- Add the vanilla extract and heavy cream and stir until everything is evenly combined.

- Grease a baking sheet with butter or oil, then spoon the batter onto the sheet in 2-inch circles, leaving at least 1 inch apart.

- Bake for 12 to 15 minutes, or until the scones are golden brown.

- Let cool on a wire rack before serving. Enjoy!

Kippers

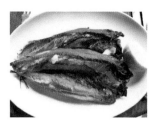

Kippers are a traditional British breakfast food. They are herring that has been split in half, cured in brine or smoked, and then cooked, usually either grilled, pan-fried or baked. Kippers have a strong aroma and slightly salty flavor. They are often served with toast or eggs for breakfast.

Ingredients:

- 2 kippers
- 2 tablespoons butter
- 1 small onion, finely chopped
- 2 tablespoons fresh parsley, finely chopped
- 2 tablespoons fresh thyme, finely chopped
- 2 teaspoons lemon juice
- Salt and pepper to taste

Instructions:

- Preheat the oven to 375F.
- Grease a shallow, oven-proof dish with the butter.
- Place the kippers in the dish, and scatter the onion over them.
- Sprinkle the parsley and thyme over the kippers and lemon juice.
- Season with salt and pepper.
- Bake in the preheated oven for 15-20 minutes, or until the kippers are cooked through and golden.
- Serve hot.

Jambalaya

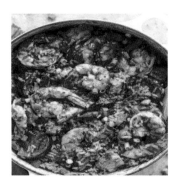

Jambalaya is a classic Creole and Cajun dish consisting of meat and/or shellfish simmered in a spicy broth with aromatic vegetables, tomatoes, and rice. Usually, jambalaya is made with a combination of meats, such as chicken, sausage, or shrimp, however, it can be made vegetarian, as well. As a hearty and flavorful one-pot meal, it is perfect for entertaining and can be served with crusty bread, a tossed salad, and a light dessert.

Ingredients:

- 1 tablespoon olive oil
- 1 green bell pepper, diced
- 1 medium onion, diced
- 3 celery stalks, diced
- 2 cloves garlic, minced
- 1 ½ teaspoon smoked paprika
- 2 teaspoons ground cumin

- ➤ 1 teaspoon dried oregano

- ➤ 1 ½ teaspoon fresh thyme

- ➤ 1 teaspoon sea salt

- ➤ 1 large pinch of cayenne pepper

- ➤ 1 can (14.5 ounces) diced tomatoes

- ➤ 2 cups vegetable broth

- ➤ 1 cup long grain brown rice

- ➤ 1 can (15.5 ounces) black-eyed peas, drained and rinsed

- ➤ 1 cup of frozen corn or okra

- ➤ 2 green onions, chopped

- ➤ Hot sauce, optional

Instructions:

- ✦ Heat oil in a large pot or Dutch oven over medium heat.

- ✦ Once hot, add in bell pepper, onion, and celery and sauté for 4-5 minutes or until the vegetables begin to soften.

- ✦ Stir in garlic, smoked paprika, cumin, oregano, thyme, sea salt, and cayenne pepper and cook an additional minute.

- ✦ Pour in tomatoes, vegetable broth, and brown rice and stir until everything is combined.

- Bring mixture to a boil, reduce heat to low and simmer, covered, for 40 minutes, stirring every 15 minutes or so.

- Once the rice is cooked through, add in black-eyed peas, corn or okra, and green onions. Stir until heated through.

- Serve jambalaya with optional hot sauce. Enjoy!

Grilled Trout

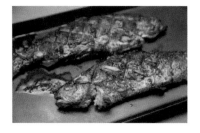

Grilled trout is a delicious main course meal typically prepared by marinating trout fillets in olive oil, garlic, and herbs such as parsley, oregano, and basil. The marinade infuses the fish with flavor, ensuring a tender and flakey end result. The marinated fillets are then cooked on an oiled, preheated grill until they are cooked through. Grilled trout has a light, delicate flavor which is enhanced by aromatic herbs and a crispy, charred skin.

Ingredients:

- ➤ 4 large trout fillets
- ➤ 1/4 cup olive oil
- ➤ 1/4 cup fresh lemon juice
- ➤ 2 teaspoons minced garlic
- ➤ 2 tablespoons finely chopped parsley
- ➤ 1 teaspoon sea salt
- ➤ 1/4 teaspoon freshly ground black pepper
- ➤ Lemon wedges for garnish

Instructions:

- ♣ Preheat your grill to medium-high heat.
- ♣ In a shallow dish, combine the olive oil, lemon juice, garlic, parsley, salt, and pepper. Add the trout fillets and turn to coat evenly with the marinade. Let the fillets marinate for at least 10 minutes.
- ♣ Grill the trout for about 4 minutes on each side or until the fillets are cooked through.
- ♣ Serve the grilled trout with lemon wedges for garnish. Enjoy!

Traditional Fish Pie

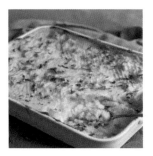

A traditional fish pie is a casserole type dish made with fish, potato, and other vegetables all combined and topped with a pastry or mashed potato layer. Typically the fish will be poached and/or flaked salmon, pollack, cod, or smoked haddock. The vegetables will usually include carrots, onions, peas, celery, and mushrooms, although any selection of vegetables may be used. The remaining ingredients often consist of seasonings like bayleaf, parsley, thyme, and a white sauce prepared with butter, flour, and milk. The pie is then topped with a pastry or mashed potato layer and baked in the oven until the top is golden brown.

Ingredients:

Filling:

- 1 lb white fish fillets (such as cod, haddock, pollock, halibut)
- 1/4 cup butter, divided
- 1 large onion, diced

- 2 cloves garlic, minced

- 2 tablespoons all- purpose flour

- 3/4 cup fish stock or vegetable stock

- 1 cup frozen peas, thawed

- 1/4 cup chopped fresh parsley

- 1 teaspoon dried thyme

- Salt and pepper, to taste

- juice of ½ lemon

Topping:

- 2 cups mashed potatoes

- 1/4 cup melted butter

- 1/4 cup grated Parmesan cheese

- 1/4 cup breadcrumbs

Instructions:

- Preheat the oven to 375 degrees F. Grease a 9x13 inch baking dish with butter.

- Heat 1 tablespoon of butter in a large skillet over medium-high heat. Once melted, add the onion and garlic. Saute until the onions are translucent and fragrant, about 5 minutes.

- Add the remaining butter to the skillet and melt. Sprinkle the flour over the onions and garlic and stir to combine. Cook for 1 minute. Slowly whisk in the stock, and bring the mixture to a simmer.

- Stir in the fish, frozen peas, parsley, thyme, salt and pepper, and lemon juice. Simmer for 5 minutes until the fish is cooked through. Transfer the mixture to the prepared baking dish.

- To make the topping, combine the mashed potatoes, melted butter, Parmesan cheese, and breadcrumbs in a bowl. Spread the mashed potatoes over the fish mixture in the dish.

- Bake in the preheated oven for 20 minutes, or until the topping is golden brown. Serve warm. Enjoy!

Lobster Bisque

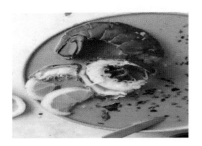

Lobster bisque is a luxurious and decadent seafood soup made with a rich and creamy seafood stock that is flavored with a combination of herbs and vegetables, including onion, celery, garlic, carrots, and white wine. The bisque is then thickened with wheat flour and cream, and chunks of lobster meat are added in for a luxurious twist. It is usually finished by swirling cream and sometimes cognac over the top, and often served with a side of croutons or crusty bread.

Ingredients:

- 2 tbsp of butter
- 2 shallots, finely chopped
- 2 carrots, finely chopped
- 2 celery stalks, finely chopped
- 2 cloves of garlic, minced
- 2 cups of dry white wine
- 6 cups of chicken broth

- 1 lb of cooked and shredded lobster meat

- ¼ tsp of cayenne pepper

- ¼ tsp of dried thyme

- ¼ tsp of white pepper

- 1 bay leaf

- 2 cups of heavy cream

- 2 tbsp of chopped fresh parsley

- Salt and pepper to taste

Instructions:

- In a large pot over medium-high heat, melt the butter and add the shallots, carrots, celery, and garlic. Cook for 5 minutes, stirring occasionally.

- Pour in the white wine and cook for 2 minutes.

- Add the chicken broth, lobster meat, cayenne pepper, thyme, white pepper, and bay leaf. Simmer for 20 minutes.

- Remove the bay leaf and transfer the soup mixture to a blender or food processor. Puree until smooth.

- Return the pureed mixture to the pot over low heat. Slowly stir in the heavy cream and parsley. Season with salt and pepper to taste.

- Simmer for 10 minutes and serve. Enjoy!

Steamed Mussels

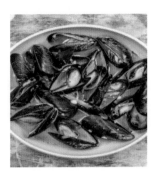

Steamed mussels are a popular dish in many countries. Commonly prepared with a light white wine or beer, garlic and herbs, the mussels are placed in a pot with a tight-fitting lid and heated until they open. They are usually served with a butter, white wine and garlic sauce. Mussels are a great low-calorie and high-protein seafood option, and they can be served on their own or with sides like crusty bread.

Ingredients:

- 2 pounds-fresh mussels
- 1 large white onion, diced
- 1 carrot, diced
- 2 stalks celery, sliced
- 2 cloves garlic, minced
- ½ cup white wine
- 2 tablespoons chopped fresh parsley

- 1 tablespoon fresh lemon juice

- Salt and freshly ground black pepper, to taste

- 2 tablespoons butter

Instructions:

- Place the mussels in a colander and rinse well under cold running water. Discard any that are open or have broken shells.

- Place a large pot over medium heat. Add the onion, carrot, celery and garlic and sauté until the vegetables are tender and lightly browned, about 8 minutes.

- Increase the heat to high and add the wine, parsley, and lemon juice. Bring the mixture to a boil, then reduce the heat to low and simmer for 5 minutes, stirring occasionally.

- Add the mussels to the pot and season with salt and pepper, to taste. Cover and cook for 8-10 minutes, or until the mussels have opened. Discard any that do not open.

- Remove the mussels from the pot and place them in bowls. Using a slotted spoon, ladle the vegetables and broth over the mussels.

- Add the butter to the broth in the pot and stir until melted. Taste and adjust the seasonings, if necessary.

↓ Serve the mussels with the melted butter sauce and crusty bread.

Enjoy!

Halibut In Parchment

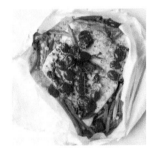

Halibut in parchment is a delicious and simple way to create a meal suited for two. The fish is seasoned with fresh herbs and spices, then wrapped in parchment paper and baked. The result is a moist, flaky, and aromatic piece of fish that's easy to serve and full of flavor. The paper packet is also easy to clean up, making, this an ideal meal for a busy night. Serve the halibut with a simple side of steamed vegetables or your favorite grain to complete the meal.

Ingredients:

- Two 5- to 6-ounce halibut fillets
- 1/2 teaspoon sea salt
- Freshly ground black pepper, to taste
- 1/4 cup dry white wine
- 1 tablespoon freshly squeezed lemon juice
- 1 tablespoon butter, cut into small pieces
- 2 tablespoons chopped fresh herbs, such as parsley, chives, tarragon, or chervil
- 2 tablespoons minced shallot
- 4 thin lemon slices

Instructions:

- Preheat oven to 425°F.
- Cut two 12-inch squares of parchment paper and set aside.
- Arrange each halibut fillet on one parchment square. Sprinkle each fillet with salt and pepper to taste.

- Combine wine, lemon juice, butter, herbs, and shallot in a small bowl. Spoon half the mixture over each fillet and top with 2 lemon slices.

- Fold the parchment around the fillet to form 4 pouches, and place on a rimmed baking sheet.

- Bake for 10 to 12 minutes, or until the packets feel firm to the touch.

- Carefully open the pouches and transfer the fish to serving plates. Spoon the remaining juices over the fish and serve.

Cod Cakes

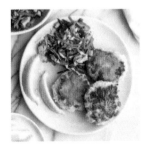

Cod cakes are a classic seafood dish made from flaked cod, mashed potatoes, and various seasonings and herbs. They are usually formed into individual patties and deep-fried until crispy and golden. They are a popular appetizer or side dish and can be served as a hearty meal with a side of salad or vegetables. They can also be found in some restaurants pre-formed and ready to fry.

Ingredients:

- ➤ 2 pounds-cod fillets, finely chopped
- ➤ ½ onion, finely chopped
- ➤ 2 tablespoons chopped fresh parsley
- ➤ 2 tablespoons freshly grated Parmesan cheese
- ➤ 2 tablespoons all-purpose flour
- ➤ 2 eggs, beaten
- ➤ 1 teaspoon dried thyme
- ➤ ½ teaspoon garlic powder
- ➤ ¼ teaspoon black pepper
- ➤ ¼ teaspoon salt
- ➤ 2 tablespoons vegetable oil

Instructions:

- ﹢ In a mixing bowl, combine the cod, onion, parsley, Parmesan, flour, eggs, thyme, garlic powder, black pepper, and salt. Mix until combined.
- ﹢ Heat the vegetable oil in a large skillet over medium heat.

- Using an ice cream scoop, scoop out the cod mixture into the skillet and flatten the balls slightly.

- Cook the cod cakes for 3-4 minutes per side, or until golden brown and crispy.

- Serve the cod cakes hot with your favorite accompaniments!

Seafood Pizza

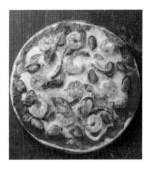

Seafood pizza is a delicious pizza pie that is topped with seafood such as shrimp, crab, or other types of fish. It may also include black olives, capers, onions, peppers, and other tasty toppings. The crust is usually thin and crispy, and the seafood is cooked before it is added to the pizza. The combination of fresh seafood and cheese make for a delicious flavor experience that is hard to beat.

Ingredients:

- ➤ 1 pizza dough (homemade or store-bought)
- ➤ 4 cloves garlic, minced
- ➤ 2 tablespoons olive oil
- ➤ 1/2 teaspoon dried oregano
- ➤ 1/4 teaspoon crushed red pepper flakes
- ➤ 1/4 teaspoon salt
- ➤ 1/4 teaspoon freshly ground black pepper
- ➤ 1/2 cup tomato sauce
- ➤ 1/2 cup shredded mozzarella cheese
- ➤ 1/2 cup cooked seafood (crab, shrimp, or scallops)
- ➤ 2 tablespoons chopped fresh parsley

Instructions:

- ↓ Preheat oven to 375 degrees F.
- ↓ In a small bowl, mix together garlic, olive oil, oregano, red pepper flakes, salt, and pepper.

- Roll out pizza dough onto a lightly floured surface. Place on a pizza pan.
- Spread tomato sauce over pizza dough. Sprinkle with mozzarella cheese.
- Top with cooked seafood.
- Bake for 20 minutes or until cheese is melted and crust is golden brown.
- Sprinkle with fresh parsley before serving. Enjoy!

Crab Cakes

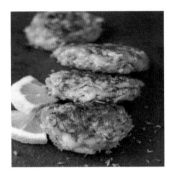

Crab cakes are a type of seafood dish that consists of minced crabmeat, breadcrumbs, eggs, and spices that are formed into cakes and pan-fried or deep-fried. They are often served with tartar sauce and a lemon wedge to bring out the sweet, salty, and savory flavors. Crab cakes are popular in the US and can be found in seafood restaurants and many home kitchens.

Ingredients:

- 1lb crabmeat
- ½ cup mayonnaise
- 2 eggs, beaten
- 1 teaspoon mustard
- ½ teaspoon Old Bay Seasoning
- ¼ teaspoon garlic powder
- 2 tablespoons of fresh parsley, minced
- 2 tablespoons of lemon juice

➢ ½ cup of Panko breadcrumbs

➢ 1 tablespoon of vegetable oil

Instructions:

+ In a large bowl, mix together the crabmeat, mayonnaise, eggs, mustard, Old Bay seasoning, garlic powder, parsley, and lemon juice.

+ Gently fold in the Panko breadcrumbs until the mixture is thoroughly combined.

+ Heat the oil in a large skillet over medium-high heat.

+ Form the crab mixture into 3-4 inch cakes and add them to the hot skillet.

+ Cook the crab cakes for 5-6 minutes per side, or until golden brown and cooked through.

+ Transfer the cooked crab cakes to a plate lined with paper towels to drain any excess oil.

+ Serve the finished crab cakes with tartar sauce, if desired. Enjoy!

Printed in Great Britain
by Amazon

38174908R00043